—— THE ——
HEALING
NETWORK
BELIEVE, RECEIVE AND MAINTAIN YOUR HEALING

THE
HEALING
NETWORK

BELIEVE, RECEIVE AND MAINTAIN YOUR HEALING

by:

MYNESHA J. ROGERS

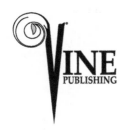

VINE PUBLISHING

Vine Publishing's name and logo are trademarks of Vine Publishing, Inc.

ISBN: 978-0-9856535-8-3 (paperback)
ISBN: 978-0-9856535-2-1 (e-book)

Library of Congress Cataloging-in-Publication Data
Library of Congress Control Number: 2020918403

Published by Vine Publishing, Inc.
New York, NY
www.vinepublish.com

Printed in the United States of America

ACKNOWLEDGEMENTS

To begin, I would like to say how humbled and honored I am that God, my Heavenly Father, has called me to encourage His people by sharing my voice through writing. I thank my Lord and Savior Jesus Christ for giving me the ability and strength to minister through this format. I thank you Lord for healing me and giving me a testimony to be a blessing to others. I give God all the glory and honor for what He is doing in and through my life!

I thank God for the people He has placed in my life. I thank my friend and publisher, Rev. Taneki Dacres, for seeing in me what I didn't see in myself and being a phenomenal midwife in the birthing of this baby. You planted the seed in me to write and I am forever grateful. You are amazing!

To my marketplace ministry coach, The Trailblazer, Carla R. Cannon, I thank you for watering that seed planted in me to write, ushering me into the belief that it can be done, and then showing me how best to begin the process. Your mentoring has been invaluable.

To my Pastors, Revs. Drs. Floyd and Elaine Flake, I thank you for being the epitome of great leadership and a shining example of authorship. You have shown me and all people across this nation how to be an extraordinary minister—one who disciples people with compassion and excellence. Your willingness to pour into us week after week, and to foster an environment for up and coming ministers to develop their ministerial gifts is truly appreciated.

To one of my spiritual mentors, Rev. Nichole Edness, I thank you for pouring into me and prophetically praying over me as I embarked upon this writing journey. I appreciate all the pearls of wisdom that you have freely shared.

To my loving Mom, my biggest cheerleader, thank you for your patience, consistent encouragement, and prayers as I took this step of faith to answer God's call and do something I never thought I could do. I love you!

To all my family and friends who have prayed for me and encouraged me along the way in this process, I thank you and I love you! You all are a big part of my healing network.

TABLE OF CONTENTS

INTRODUCTION

I f you take a moment to reflect on your life and what's happening in the world today, you may notice that there seems to be more people suffering from one ailment or the other. Whether it's high blood pressure and diabetes, or more severe diseases like lupus or cancer—it seems each one of us knows someone who is dealing with sickness. In fact, you may have a family member or friend who has not experienced healing and is constantly spending exorbitant amounts of money on prescription pills just to survive. Or, you may be the one struggling with sickness for some time and can't seem to find relief from the symptoms. I don't know about you, but for me, it's very disheartening to see so many people suffering.

Almost every week, I receive a call to pray for someone who received an unfavorable diagnosis, or who is about to undergo surgery, or worse, someone nearing the end of life due to sickness. What's more, as I write this book, the world is currently facing a major pandemic—an aggressively-contagious disease called the Coronavirus, also known as COVID-19. As I pen these words, I am sad to say that hundreds of thousands of people around the world have been hospitalized because of COVID-19, and sadly thousands have died. It's in these times that some people tend to ask the question, "Does God still heal today?" or "Is it God's will for all to be healed?" Have you ever questioned God's power and/ or desire to heal? Have you been struggling with sickness and are wondering when you'll be healed? Have you witnessed family and friends suffer for years, and you are wondering if their healing will ever manifest? If you have wrestled with any of these questions, then this book is for you. Know that God has the power to heal, and it is His desire for you and your loved one to be made whole.

As long as I can remember, I have always despised being sick. Whether it was a simple cold or the flu, or a chronic illness, I hated being sick, and I hated seeing others sick. It was this disdain toward sickness that produced a passion within to see all people healed and whole. While I have witnessed and heard inspiring testimonies about God doing great things through people who are disabled and/or ill, I still choose to believe that sickness is not from God. I still believe that the work Jesus did by dying for us on the cross has destroyed the power of all sickness and disease. Why do I emphatically believe this? Well, because I am a living witness to the healing power of God. He has healed me and I have witnessed God's healing in the lives of loved ones.

In this book, I share my testimony and the testimonies of family and friends. You will learn the importance of a holistic approach to believing, receiving, and maintaining your healing. This holistic approach includes a network of beliefs, principles, people, tools, strategies, and practices. A network is "an interconnected or interrelated chain, group, or system." The Healing Network is an interconnection of faith, action, and relationships (The F.A.R. Principle). It is my belief and experience that all these components are necessary for optimal health. Grounded on Bible principles, each chapter of this book presents an in-depth exploration of The

F.A.R. Principle.

The Healing Network provides you with practical steps to help you obtain and maintain healing, so that you may live the abundant life God wants you to have. As you read this book, it is my prayer that you will know, without a doubt, that it is God's will for you to be healed, and that healing is readily available to you if you believe, and effectively operate your network.

Now, at this point, let me confess that I grappled with whether this was the right time to release this book, especially when so many have been affected and infected by COVID-19. I'm sensitive to the fact that you may be finding it difficult to believe in God's healing power. Given the current climate, to declare that God wants you to be healed is a bold statement. You may find it difficult to believe because you have witnessed your friends and loved ones succumb to the disease. I get it. But I still believe, and you should too. The fact is, as much as we have witnessed the devastating impact of the virus, we have also witnessed the healing power of God. Yes, some died, but many more survived and were healed. I still believe that God is a Healer even in the midst of His sovereign decision to allow disease—a decision that we don't always understand. God has healed and is still healing amid this world crisis. That means that healing is always possible, and we should continue to seek it and expect it. Jesus said, all things are possible for those who believe (Mark 9:23). So, believe, and let's begin exploring the Healing Network!

Believe

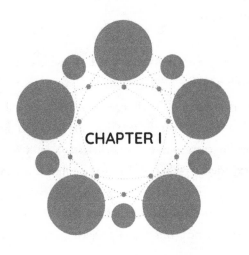

CHAPTER I

Does God Really Want You Healed?

Jesus Christ is the same yesterday and today and forever.

— Hebrews 13:8 (NIV)

E very decision we make in life starts with a belief. If we decide to go to school, it is because we believe that education leads to more opportunities and a better life. If we decide to apply for a particular job, it is because we believe that job will provide an income and perhaps, a sense of purpose. If we decide to get married, it is because we believe we are in love and are compatible with that person. When we make the decision to follow Jesus Christ and receive the gift of salvation, it's because we believe Jesus is the Son of God who lived, died, resurrected, and is the way to eternal life. So, why is it that many of us struggle with unbelief as it relates to healing?

Belief is important for all aspects of life, especially when it comes to healing. We must believe that God heals and that healing is possible for every one of us. Belief starts with a conviction through experience or knowledge that a thing is achievable and obtainable. As Christians, we know that faith comes by hearing and hearing by the Word of God (Rom. 10:17), and as such, we can believe that God wants us to be healed because it is written in His Word.

Since the beginning of time, God created us as whole beings. We were made in God's image and likeness, lacking nothing, with the ability to live life eternally healthy and whole. Due to the disobedience of the first man and woman (Genesis 3), the curse of death came upon humankind. This curse not only separated us from the Creator, but it also opened the door to sin, sickness, and disease. With the fall of humanity, God, in His love for His creation, decided to send His only begotten son, Jesus, to redeem us from the curse and reconcile us to a fruitful relationship with Him. So, what does this all mean for us? It means when we place our faith in Jesus, we are not only in right standing with God, the Father, but we are also the recipients of God's blessings, which include forgiveness of all our sins and healing from all our diseases (Psalm 103:2-3). So, does God want us to be healed? Of course He does. He desires for us to be made whole (1 Thessalonians 5:23). God is concerned about the things that concern us (Psalm 138:8), and if sickness is our concern, then our loving God is concerned. God wants us to be healed yesterday, today, and forevermore. He healed in years past, He's healing today, and will heal forever (Hebrews 13:8).

YESTERDAY

Whether we realize it or not, God has always revealed Himself as the God who heals. Throughout the Bible, from the Old Testament to the New Testament, God has shown Himself faithful to His people. He was faithful to heal King Abimelech when Abraham prayed for him (Gen. 20:17). He was faithful to comfort the children of Israel when He declared, "I am the Lord who heals you." (Exodus 15:26). He was faithful to speak through King Solomon in Proverbs 4:20–22, when he declared "...Pay attention to what I say; turn your ear to my words. Do not let them out of your sight, keep them within your heart; for they are life to those who find them and health to one's whole body" (NIV). God was faithful to heal through Levitical Priests. He was faithful to speak through prophets like Isaiah who declared that our Savior, "*was* wounded for our transgressions, *He was* bruised for our iniquities; the chastisement for our peace *was* upon Him, and by His stripes we are healed" (Isaiah 53:5 NKJV). God has proven Himself to be faithful, and it is not only His desire for us to be healed, but He also sent His Word to heal us.

Jesus, the Son of the living God, was the Word wrapped in flesh. Fully divine and fully human, God, through His Son dwelt

among us, and while on earth He preached, taught and healed. "...
Jesus went about all Galilee, teaching in their synagogues, preach-
ing the gospel of the kingdom, and healing all kinds of sickness
and all kinds of disease among the people" (Matthew 4:23 NKJV).
Blind eyes were opened at His touch, the lame walked, the mute
spoke, the tormented received deliverance at His command—
wherever Jesus went, people were healed. His power, coupled with
the faith of the people, manifested healing. God healed through
His power, love, and through His Son. He healed yesterday, and
He is healing us today.

TODAY

"Surely he took up our pain and bore our suffering, yet we
considered him punished by God, stricken by him, and afflicted.
But he was pierced for our transgressions, he was crushed for our
iniquities; the punishment that brought us peace was on him, and
by his wounds we are healed" (Isaiah 53:4–5 NIV). Surely, Jesus
took up our pain and bore our suffering. Surely, Jesus was pierced
for our transgressions. Surely, Jesus was crushed for our iniquities.
Surely by Jesus' wounds, we are healed today. This is the finished
work of the cross. When we consider whether healing is available
to us today, we must look to the cross. It was on the cross that Jesus
paid the ultimate price for us all. It was on the cross—beaten, tor-
tured, battered, disgraced, crucified, that Jesus, the sacrificial Lamb
of God, shed His blood so that we can be delivered, healed and
made whole today. Before the cross, we were all doomed—des-

tined to live in sin, sickness and despair. But God, in His unfailing love for us, sacrificed His Son in the ultimate redemptive act. We were redeemed from the penalty of sin, and brought back into right relationship with God. The cross restored us to God's original plan for us—the same plan He had when Adam and Eve lived in the Garden of Eden. It is His plan that we would have full access to Him, and that we would live victoriously on earth—forgiven of our sins, free from sickness, and living the abundant life.

So, does God want us to be healed today? We can look to the cross and His Word and answer with a huge YES. The prophet Isaiah prophesied it and Jesus fulfilled it. By His wounds, we are healed. The scripture does not say, we may be healed. Or, we could be healed; or sometimes, we are healed. It says, we ARE healed. That's the finished work of Jesus; that's the healing power of our Savior. He broke the power of sin, and gave us victory over the curses of the original sin, of which sickness is one of the curses. (Deuteronomy 28:22). Today, we can ask God to manifest His healing in us. Today, we can receive healing! Today, by faith, we can be made whole, now and forever more. Why? Because He got up.

FOREVER

Forever means continually, incessantly, always—lasting for an endless period of time ~ without ever ending; eternally.[1] By His stripes we are eternally free, and forever healed. The finished work is not based solely on the suffering and death of our Savior, but also on the fact that we have an everlasting victory through the resurrection of our Lord. Jesus got up. In His resurrection was the "moral recovery of spiritual truth."[2] His resurrection allows us to grab a hold of God's truth—of His promise that although Adam's sin brought death (moral, spiritual and physical) to us all, Jesus' death brought us back to life (1 Corinthians 15:21). That, my dear friends is the recovery of spiritual truth.

Jesus was resurrected from death and is now seated at the right hand of the Father in heaven (Luke 22:69). Because He lives, we are redeemed forever. Because He lives, generations who are saved and believe are forever healed. No matter what life brings and heath challenges we may face, we can believe for healing, and expect God to heal. The reality is we may experience seasons of ailment, but even in those seasons, we can and must believe God for healing. God is not a man that He should lie, or a son of man that He should repent (Numbers 23:19). If He said it, it is so...and He said, by His wounds we are, and forever will be, healed. Keep the faith, pray without ceasing, believe God, and always expect to be healed.

How does the Word of God affirm God's desire
for you to be healed?

_____

_____

_____

_____

_____

_____

_____

_____

_____

_____

_____

_____

_____

_____

_____

_____

_____

_____

_____

_____

_____

Receive

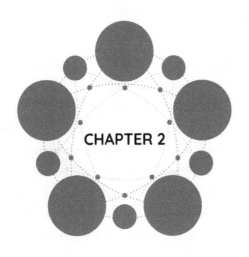

CHAPTER 2

Prayer, the Greatest Tool of Faith!

Therefore I tell you, whatever you ask for in prayer, believe that you have received it, and it will be yours. — Mark 11:24 (NIV)

It was a summer morning in 1991, when I woke up and quickly realized I could not move my wrist. It was the strangest feeling I had ever felt, and it frightened me. I could not understand why this was happening. Prior to going to bed, I did not have any pain, discomfort, or feel sick. There were no warning signs leading to this alarming moment. Immediately, I called for my mom to explain what I was experiencing and she took me to the emergency room. After the doctors examined me, they could not figure out why I was experiencing these symptoms, so they prescribed muscle relaxers, believing that it would solve the problem. The following days, my joints were still stiff, and in addition, I began experiencing pain and dark spots appearing on my legs. The muscle relaxers were ineffective, so I decided to visit my primary physician.

Unfortunately, she was also unable to help me. I was so confused by this sudden ailment and I needed answers. Finally, my mom took me to the hospital where she worked, and it was there that the doctors referred me to a rheumatologist, who then diagnosed me with a mild case of lupus. At that very moment I thought to myself, "What? How could this be?" This was not something I was familiar with or had heard much about. In addition, to discover there wasn't a cure was very traumatic for me. I wanted answers. "How did I get lupus?" But the doctors had no definitive answers. All I was told was, "We're not sure," or "There are different things that can trigger it." Have you ever been there? Have you ever been diagnosed with a condition that your doctors could not explain? It is such a frustrating and scary situation.

I was placed on steroids and aspirin to control my symptoms. To avoid triggering the symptoms, I was told not to spend too much time in the sun, and to wear sunblock all the time. It was also necessary for me to get sufficient rest and avoid stress. My life changed in an instant. Arthritic pain and spots on my lower legs seemed like it would be my new norm. *Me?!* I thought. *Me, the one who could not tolerate having a simple cold, how could I be diagnosed with a serious autoimmune disease that is incurable?* This was so hard to believe. It was a disheartening diagnosis. However, *something* in me could not accept that I would have a debilitating disease for the rest of my life. After getting over the scare of this event, I went on living. I did what I could to make sure I didn't trigger any more symptoms. I stayed out of the sun and took the medication.

After several months, the symptoms started to subside and I began to declare that I would be healed in spite of the diagnosis. I started developing a stronger relationship with my Lord and Savior Jesus Christ through prayer. I became more aware of His healing power through the preached word, and I began praying the Word of God over my situation. I don't quite remember exactly when it clicked for me but I decided not to accept this diagnosis and continued to wholeheartedly seek God in prayer, asking for His healing and speaking God's truth over my life. I declared that by Jesus' stripes, I would be healed.

About a year after the diagnosis, I was no longer experiencing symptoms of pain or bruise marks on my skin, and I was feeling good. My rheumatologist took me off the medication but still advised me to get sufficient rest and stay out of the sun for long periods of time. I believed I was healed. Now, with all transparency, I must say that doubt crept up from time to time, but each time it did I would quickly dismiss it and continue to declare my healing. Doctors could not explain why I was no longer experiencing the symptoms of lupus, but all I know is that I was once sick but now I am healed! I felt better and knew within my heart that I was healed! I know because it has been over twenty-four years since that diagnosis, and I am still healed. To God be the glory!

You may have been diagnosed with an unfathomable ailment. You may be at your lowest point, weighed down by a sickness, but continue to keep the faith. Keep praying. Keep believing. Faith is the key but it must be accompanied with action, and prayer is the first action step towards healing. Prayer is communication with God our Creator, through Jesus Christ, our Savior. Philippians 4:6 exhorts us: "Do not worry about anything, but in everything by prayer and supplication with thanksgiving let your requests be made known to God" (NRSV). It is in prayer that we commune with God about our challenges, express how we feel, and ask God's blessings to manifest in our lives, but prayer is not only making requests—it is also reminding Him of His promises for our lives. Prayer is claiming what God said we could have—claiming His gift of healing. It's in declaring the scriptures, God's Word, back to Him in prayer.

In his book called *The Believer's Authority*, the late Bro. Kenneth E. Hagin, who had an effective healing ministry, said the following about meditating on scripture prayers: "Learn to pray them for yourself. Feed on their truths until they become a part of your inner consciousness. Then they will dominate your life. But don't try to accept them mentally; you've got to get the revelation of them in your spirit." [3] Pray God's Word, but I implore you to go beyond reciting the Word of God. As you pray God's Word, allow your inner consciousness to connect with what's flowing from your lips. Pray with your soul and let the Word quicken your spirit. It is in this moment that what's been hidden is revealed, and it is through divine revelation that faith grows. It is the prayer offered in faith that will make the sick well (James 5:5). Prayer wrapped in faith is our first action step towards wholeness. I believed God and prayed His promises over my life and situation. It does not matter what any person says, or what the doctors say, or even what we say to ourselves, what matters is what the Word of God says. When we exercise our faith through prayer, we will see the manifestation of healing in our lives.

It was on the cross that Jesus took all our diseases, and by His stripes we are healed (Isaiah 53:4). I am healed, and I believe that what God has done for me, He is willing to do for you. Prayer changes things. I am a witness to the power of communing with God. It was through the power of prayer, coupled with faith-filled works, that I received victory and overcame health challenges. But, I am also a witness of the power of prayer working in the lives of family and friends. Prayer works, and the following testimonies are proof of its power.

MY AUNT'S STORY

My aunt, Diana, was my mom's youngest sibling. She was the aunt who baby-sat my brother and me when we were younger. More than any other aunt, Diana was the one who played with the children of the family. A big kid at heart, Diana was the one who liked teasing everyone, who had the energy to run after everyone at the end of every family gathering to get the last tag. But, like some people from her generation, she was a smoker. She was not just a social smoker, but she smoked daily. Eventually, the smoking took a toll on her body. Things began to change for this youthful, playful woman. Aunt Diana started to slow down. It became difficult for her to breath.

Although breathing became difficult for my aunt, she had a hard time kicking the smoking habit. Her condition grew worse, and one day after finding it extremely difficult to breath, she went to the emergency room. Diana was diagnosed with lung cancer and pneumonia, and the family was devastated. As the doctors prepared for surgery to remove the cancer, they asked her the question that no likes to be asked: "If something was to happen during surgery, should we resuscitate?" My aunt responded, "Do all that they can to keep me alive!" And with that, Diana was wheeled into surgery.

The family was relieved and happy when Diana made it through the surgery. Hope was restored and we all expected it to be a smooth recovery, but that was not the case. In fact, Aunt Diana had a difficult time recovering. The doctors had to put her on a respirator three times, but her condition grew worse. Her organs began to shut down, and the family was once again called to the hospital. Unfortunately, my mom and I, along with another aunt and cousins, were out of town. The doctors believed that Aunt Diana was nearing the end of life, and we were once again devastated. Unable to predict the timing of her demise but certain of her declining condition, one minute the doctors told the family who were present at hospital that she would not make it through the day, and the next minute they informed them that she only had a few hours to live. As my uncle relayed the doctors' reports to us, we felt an overwhelming sadness, as we were not sure if we would make it back home in time to see her alive. I was dumbfounded and could not receive the negative report. I did not want to believe this was happening to my 63-year-young, fun-loving aunt who still had many years of life ahead of her.

We made it back in time to visit my aunt in the ICU as she hung on for dear life. As I looked at her swollen body, I still refused to accept that death would have its final say, and that's when we did what we knew best...we prayed. As we gathered together around my aunt's bed, holding hands, I laid one hand on my aunt and we prayed the "Lord's Prayer" (Matt. 6:9–13). With holy boldness, I prayed believing and declaring she would be healed. As we walked away from her bed, the nurse said to me, "We'll see." I thought to myself, *what a negative response to say to a family who chose to believe in the power of prayer*. But, with a determined spirit of faith, I emphatically responded, "Yes, we will see!" And sure enough, God answered our prayers, for the prayers of the righteous avails much (James 5:16). God truly allowed us to see a miracle, for the next day we received a call from my uncle saying, "Guess who is awake and talking?!" Overnight, things turned for the better and the condition of my aunt's organs began to improve.

Aunt Diana was moved from ICU to a regular room where she continued to receive treatment. She was put on a breathing tracheotomy and was treated with oxygen. As her lungs became stronger and her energy increased, she was transferred to a rehabilitation facility. After several weeks in the rehabilitation facility, the breathing tracheotomy was removed and my aunt was taken off of oxygen. Her condition improved daily, and not long after, Diana was released from rehab. She was breathing on her own! This was such an awe-inspiring experience.

To witness my aunt walk out of rehab on her own, with no oxygen, was the manifestation of God's healing through the power of prayer. In spite of what it looked like—in spite of the reports, in spite of what the doctors said, in spite of the fact that death was knocking at her door, through faith and prayer, Aunt Diana not only walked out of the hospital, but she also lived another four years, enjoying her life and time with her family. God is truly good, and I believe that our prayers on behalf of the infirmed are heard by the loving, merciful God. I was humbled and honored to have been there to witness this miraculous healing, and I know that God is still healing us today.

You may know someone dealing with an ailment. It may be your family member, friend or even an associate. Pray for that person. Pray in faith knowing that God hears you. Pray and continue to pray for their healing. In spite of what it looks like, pray without ceasing (1 Thessalonians 5:17).

SHARON'S STORY

One evening after a small Bible study and fellowship at my home, my friend Sharon shared that doctors had diagnosed her with having a microprolactinoma, which is a benign tumor of the pituitary gland that produces an excess amount of the hormone *prolactin*. Since the tumor was benign, there was no need for any treatment. Her doctor would monitor its activity, to make sure there was no growth. Sharon was scheduled to go back to her doctor that coming week for a follow-up visit, so before she left my home that night, I felt the need to pray with her. I asked my other friend who was present at the Bible study to join us in prayer. We prayed that she would be healed of this tumor and that she would receive a good report from the doctor. A week later Sharon contacted me to say that God answered our prayers. When she went back to the doctor to get the results of the exam, the doctor informed her that not only was there no growth, but that there was no tumor found! My reaction was, "Wow, glory to God!" Sharon was healed! Her situation was yet again a reminder that prayer still works and God still heals.

A FEW MORE TESTIMONIES

Over the years, I have witnessed God's healing power manifest in the lives of others through prayer. While visiting a friend at her church, I prayed for a young lady suffering from a headache. The pain was so bad that she found it difficult to enjoy the event, so out of compassion for her, I laid hands on her and prayed for the headache to leave her. After that prayer, a little while later, the young lady said she was no longer experiencing pain. On another occasion, I prayed for a friend who was suddenly experiencing back pain. A few hours later after I prayed, she revealed to me that the pain in her back was gone. Glory be to God!

I am grateful that I was able to witness God's healing power manifest in the lives of others. Although, I can't say that I have witnessed the manifestation of healing in every individual for whom I have prayed, I can say without a doubt that healing is possible. So, be not discouraged, but pray. God is no respecter of persons (Acts 10:34); if He heard my prayers, He hears your prayers. We can rest in Him and have peace in our circumstances knowing that He sees, He knows and He cares. God wants us to live healed and whole lives, but the reality is that sometimes there are things blocking us from receiving His promises. Prayer is essential and it is in our time spent with the sovereign God that He will reveal any mountain erected in our lives that blocks us from walking in divine healing.

Recall a time when you witnessed the power of prayer

_____

_____

_____

_____

_____

_____

_____

_____

_____

_____

_____

_____

_____

_____

_____

_____

_____

_____

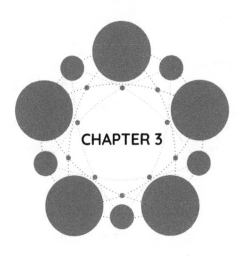

CHAPTER 3

Mountains In Our Way

*For assuredly, I say to you, whoever says to this mountain, 'Be removed
and be cast into the sea,' and does not doubt in his heart, but believes
that those things he says will be done, he will have whatever he says.*
— Mark 11:23 (NKJV)

A mountain is "a landmass that projects conspicuously above its
surroundings and is higher than a hill; or it's a great mass."[4]
In life's journey, a mountain may seem intimidating and insur-
mountable. It is a blockage separating us from our desired destiny.
Many of us are crying out to the Lord for healing, but we have yet
to receive it. Some of us are in the valley of sickness, but there is
a huge mountain standing between us and our promised land—a

land flowing with health and wholeness. Mountains are in our way, blocking and preventing us from receiving all that God has for us. These mountains may be unforgiveness, stress, fear, negative thinking and negative speaking. These mountains are not divinely erected, and they do not suddenly appear, but they are blockages that gradually grow.

A lack of forgiveness, stress, fear, and/or negativity are great masses that are erected in our lives and keep us from seeing what's ahead of us, making it difficult for us to move forward. However, God reminds us that if we have faith, we can speak to our mountains, and they will be removed (Mark 11:23). If you are tired of being sick and tired, then it's time to speak to some mountains.

UNFORGIVENESS

In June 2017, Essence Magazine issued an online article titled, "Forgive! Why Your Life Could Depend On It." Focused on how unforgiveness can affect our health adversely, the writer of this article, Gina Roberts-Grey, wrote "animosity, resentment and an inability or unwillingness to forgive prompt that same cascade of hormonal and physical feedback as when you're faced with something dangerous or scary. Whenever you revisit that anger and bitterness, you flip on your fight or flight reflex."[5] Mrs. Roberts-Grey also shared a quote from Meryl B. Rome, M.D., the owner of Boca Integrative Health in Boca Raton, Florida which describes what happens to a person when they are in a continuous state of distraught. Dr. Rome said, "You'll have an increase in heart rate and blood pressure and sugar in your bloodstream."[5]

Unforgiveness is an emotional mountain that keeps us in a valley of anger and bitterness. It is in this valley that we hold on to our hurt feelings—we nurture our wounds and open the doors to ailments. Unforgiveness is a mountain that blocks us from intimacy with God. When we hold onto grudges—what he did or what she did—when we refuse to let go of offenses and forgive, whether or not we recognize it, our hearts become hardened, and a hardened heart is not receptive towards God. God desires intimacy—a deeper relationship with you, but the Word of God is clear that He also requires us to show mercy and grace...to forgive.

In Matthew 18:21-22, Peter, Jesus' disciple, asked Him, "Lord, how often shall my brother sin against me, and I forgive him? Up to seven times?" Jesus' response was, "I do not say to you, up to seven times, but up to seventy times seven." Wow! Many of us find it difficult to forgive once, but Jesus said we are to forgive seventy times seven. In other words, we are to forgive and keep on forgiving. Now I know this may be difficult for some of you to accept. You may be saying, "Well, this person hurt me so bad, they don't deserve my forgiveness." Or, you may be thinking, "I can't forgive them, it's too hard to do it." I know it's hard, but God does not require anything from us that He has not equipped us to do.

We can gain the strength to forgive by simply looking at Jesus' sacrifice on the cross. It was while hanging on a wooden cross, suffering, enduring agonizing pain at the hands of people, that He interceded for humanity and asked the Father to forgive us all (Luke

23:34). Surely, if Jesus can forgive us, you can forgive every person who has hurt you. God has already given you the strength and power to forgive. In fact, 2 Timothy 1:7 says, "For God did not give us a spirit of cowardice, but rather a spirit of power and of love and of self-discipline" (NRSV). God's Spirit is within you, and it's His Spirit that empowers you to forgive—to love the person who mistreated you, to love as Christ loved. It is His Spirit within you that empowers you to have a disciplined mind—a mind that is not focused on the hurt, but one that focuses on seeing the best in others. God's Spirit empowers us to forgive, and it is in the release that we ourselves are released from the pain of the past—from our bondages, and free to overcome any mountain erected in our way. Forgive, and may the healing rivers flow as you surrender it all to God.

STRESS

In a 2012 report issued by the American Psychological Association (APA) titled "The Impact of Stress", the question was asked, "Is 'stressed out' the new normal?" In the report, they referenced a survey called, *Stress in America*. This survey reported that many Americans consistently experience extreme levels of stress. Measuring with a 10-point scale, 10 being the highest level of stress, it was reported that twenty percent of the Americans surveyed had stress levels at 8, 9 or 10. In addition, in their most recent survey published in early 2017, the APA highlighted how technology and social media are now major triggers of stress.[6] As I read these reports, I thought about the fact that there are many triggers that cause us to experience stress, and the reality is that stress has the ability to cause emotional and even physical harm to our bodies. Think about it. Have you ever noticed a stressed-out individual rubbing their head, or suddenly having a migraine? Have you ever noticed that some people develop stomach aches when they become extremely worried? Stress takes a toll on a person's body, which may result in illnesses such as high blood pressure, stomach ulcers, and rash outbreaks. Stress, if not managed and/or subdued, may result in dis-ease.

In the times we're living in, with increased evil in the world—mass murders, economic downturns, increase in unjust arrests and incarceration, as well as the frightening political state of affairs of this nation under unstable leadership—there is no wonder why more and more people are experiencing stress. The average cares of life—lack of income, loss of loved ones, troubling relationships, striving for success—are enough to weigh us down and have us "stressed out." Are you worrying about your family members and friends? Are you worrying about how you will make ends meet? The Word of God reminds us, "Do not worry about anything, but in everything by prayer and supplication make your requests known to God" (Philippians 4:6 NRSV). Now, you may be thinking, "That's easier said than done," but there is nothing you cannot do with God's strength and Spirit guiding you.

Philippians 4:6–7 reminds us to keep the faith, to give our cares to the Lord, and to trust Him to provide all our needs. The

Pauline text highlights three stress-busting methods: prayer, supplication and thanksgiving. *"Do not worry about anything, but in everything by prayer and supplication make your requests known to God..."* Paul exhorts us to talk to God—to earnestly, seriously, and with intent, talk to God about everything. We can trust our loving God with our secrets and concerns. Talk with God, but the texts also remind to make our requests to Him. No one can do for us what God can. What are you in need of? Tell God. Let your needs and wants be made known to Him. What are your specific requests? These are your supplications. Give all your cares over to God, and while you are doing so, thank Him in advance.

Thanksgiving is an act of faith, and faith pleases God. Thank God for miracles. Thank God for healing your body and mind. Thank God, for "who can add an hour to their life by worrying?" (Luke 12:25). Worrying causes us to become sick—suddenly, our blood pressure is raised, and age lines are more evident. Suddenly we don't look youthful as we once did, or feel energized because stress and worry slowly drains us. But God is your source and your resource. *"Do not worry about anything, but in everything by prayer and supplication make your requests known to God..."* and His strength, His healing, His peace will destroy every mountain of stress.

THE SPIRIT OF FEAR

I didn't know what was happening, but I knew something was wrong. *Why am I feeling like this?* I sat there, hands on chest, wondering if the burning, tightening and aches down my arm was a heart attack. *This could not be happening,* I thought. Not wanting to take a chance, I made my way to the hospital. Little did I know this would be a recurring event. Life has a way of throwing us curved balls and causing disruptions. I could not have imagined being admitted to the hospital three times within two months with symptoms that mimicked a heart attack. I was not sure what was happening, and neither did the doctors. The good news was that I had not had a heart attack, and test after test revealed that my heart was, in fact, in good condition. I admit, I had a sense of relief but, I must also admit that deep within, I worried that it might happen again. Why? Because the doctors could not provide a clear diagnosis. That state of uncertainty caused me to worry, but then I had to remind myself to go to The Source of life—to God, our Creator. It was while hospitalized and seeking God's wisdom that the Spirit of God revealed the root of the anxiety I was feeling. God revealed that fear was the underlying culprit.

God has not given us a spirit of fear, but of power and of love and of a sound mind (2 Timothy 1:7). Fear is not of God, and it is a doorway that invites the enemy to attack our minds and bodies. Stress and worry occur when our focus is on the cares of life instead of our Source of life. Stress and worry are rooted in fear—fear of lack, fear of failure, fear of loss, fear for our loved one's well-being, and fear of the unknown. Mark 6:5-6a says, "Now He could do no mighty work there, except that He laid His hands on a few sick people and healed *them.* And He marveled because of their unbelief" (NKJV). Fear is unbelief in God's power and promises. It is a mighty mountain that blocks us from seeing God's goodness. It is the mountain that the enemy erects in our minds when we are faced with a negative diagnosis. Fear makes us think the worst, "Will I relapse? Will it get worse? Will I die? Fear's attempt is to grip and hold us in a place of negativity. But I encourage you to replace fear with faith. Meditate on God's promises. Remind yourself of God's love. Renew your mind daily. When the disciples were caught in a tumultuous storm, Jesus said, "Why are you so afraid? Do you still have no faith?" (Mark 4:40 NIV). Today, Jesus is asking you the same question, "Why are you so afraid?" Today, decide to demolish that mountain of fear and move confidently towards your healing.

NEGATIVE THINKING AND SPEAKING

In February 2017, the Mayo Clinic issued an Internet article titled, "Positive Thinking: Stop Negative Self-Talk to Reduce Stress." The focus of this article was the effects of positive thinking on a person's mental and physical health. What was discovered was that a person's health is affected by how he or she views life, whether from an optimistic or pessimistic point of view. According to the article, positive thinking has health benefits such as, "Greater resistance to the common cold; better psychological and physical well-being; better cardiovascular health and reduced risk of death from cardiovascular disease."[7] On the other hand, it is then safe to say that negative thinking negatively affects our bodies. So, how have you been thinking?

The Word of God tells us that when we meditate on positive things, we can have peace. Philippians 4:8 says, "Finally, brethren, whatever things are true, whatever things *are* noble, whatever things *are* just, whatever things *are* pure, whatever things *are* lovely, whatever things *are* of good report, if *there is* any virtue and if *there is* anything praiseworthy—meditate on these things" (NKJV). We are what we think about (Proverbs 23:7) and if we desire to be made whole, then we must first renew our minds (Romans 12:2). You may have heard that the battlefield is in the mind, and guess what? It is!

It is the devil's tactic to bombard our minds with negativity. He spreads lies in an effort to counteract the work of God in our lives. The devil is a liar and the father of lies (John 8:44). He plants seeds of doubt and fear in our minds, hoping we would forget God's promises. It is his hope that we would give up and never become who God wants us to be. He is indeed a liar, but we as believers can rejoice in knowing God has given us the tools and strategies to counteract every evil dart. So, how do we get rid of negative thinking and maintain a positive mindset?

According to the Mayo Clinic article, "Positive thinking often starts with self-talk." What are you saying to yourself? What are you speaking about your situation? We can counteract negative thinking by what we speak. Proverbs 18:21 says, "Death and life *are* in the power of the tongue: and they that love it shall eat the fruit thereof" (KJV). What fruit are your words bearing? Speak life. If we want to be "stress-free", we have to speak it. If we want to think positively, we have to speak positively. If we want to be healed, we have to speak healing! We will have whatever we say, if we believe (Mark 11:23). Our negative words and thinking are mountains blocking us from a healthy, whole life. As creation, made in the image of the Creator, we are to do what the Creator has done. God spoke existence into being, and we have the power to speak into being our healing. Speak life!

Whether you have mountains of unforgiveness, stress, fear, negative thinking and speaking, or other types of mountains in your life, speak the Word of God to those mountains. Command those mountains to leave your life, in the name of Jesus. See the mountains moving—believe God and it shall be done. Speak what God says, but do your part to receive and maintain your healing.

What mountains can you identify that have been in the way of your healing?

_____

_____

_____

_____

_____

_____

_____

_____

_____

_____

_____

_____

_____

_____

_____

_____

_____

_____

_____

_____

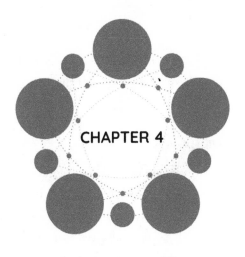

CHAPTER 4

O' Taste and See

*In the same way, faith by itself, if it is not accompanied by action,
is dead.. —* James 2:17 (NIV)

T hus far, we have delved into the spiritual side of the Healing
Network. We have talked about the importance of faith,
prayer, moving mountains, and positive thinking and speaking,
but now it's time to discuss some of the practical steps we can take
to transform our health and lives. When action accompanies faith,
we have a winning formula. Faith without action is dead (James
2:17), so in order to receive and maintain healing, we must take
the necessary steps. These steps may include making wise decisions
about what we feed our bodies. It may also include changing our

level of physical activity. While I believe in divine healing, in many situations, healing occurs through proper nutrition, rest, and exercise.

BACK TO THE BASICS

We are what we eat, and to experience healing one of the first things we can do is to go back to genesis—back to the beginning. In Genesis 1:29–30, God gave the first man (Adam) and woman (Eve) every seed-bearing fruit and green plant for food. Notice that God's first food supply to his creation was plant-based. God provided fruit and green plant for consumption, and I believe that good health starts with our eating habits. It was not until after the flood in Genesis 9 that God introduced humanity to animal food sources. While we are not sure why God allowed Noah and his family to eat meat, what we know for sure is that plant-based foods supply the body with alkalinity, while animal meat supplies acidity. As such, we can surmise that a healthy body requires a balance of both alkaline and acidic foods. In fact, according to an October 2018 article titled, "Alkaline Water: Beneficial or All Hype?", Rachael Link, Registered Dietician, informs that on a scale between 0–14, an individual's pH levels on average should be approximately a 7.365, which means the blood would have a 60/40 alkaline-to-acid ratio.[8] While the 60 represents more plant-based foods, there is still need for the 40—the animal-based foods. According to the above ratio, more plant-based consumption is the key.

Now, when I speak of "diet", I'm not referring to a temporary restriction from certain foods. When I speak of diet, I'm referring to a healthy eating lifestyle. Diets that are majority alkaline are vegan-based diets. On my journey towards healing, I chose a vegan-based diet. I also participated in a five-day juice fast to detox my body, which resulted in relief from inflammation and allowed more flexibility in my joints. When I chose vegetables over meat, I lost weight and regulated my blood pressure. I know the importance of an alkaline-based diet, and while it may not be for everyone, I do believe that eating more alkaline foods than acidic foods will result in a healthier lifestyle. I do believe that more plants in our diets may be the medication we need to heal our bodies from diseases. We eat to live and not live to eat, and no one knows this better than my friend, nutritionist, Fabienne Volel Keller. It was Fabienne who introduced me to a plant-based diet. Her help and guidance led me to a healthier lifestyle, so it was important for me to include her expertise in this area.

ALTERNATIVE MEDICINE FROM FABIENNE VOLEL KELLER, NUTRITIONIST

Fabienne Volel Keller has been a nutritionist for the past ten years, working for the New York State Department of Health, as well as various New York City hospitals as a clinical nutritionist and consultant. In addition, Fabienne facilitates workshops on nutrition in the New York City area. Passionate about helping people live their best lives through healthy eating, she uses spiritual insights and practical steps to help facilitate healing. As I consulted Fabienne for this book, she told me about the many revelations God gave her regarding the relationship between what we consume and our health. God revealed to Fabienne that, "If man ate what God provided for us to eat to nourish the body—in the way He provided it, instead of what we created by altering it—there wouldn't be so many diseases." But one of Fabienne's "aha" revelations, and one that had me in awe, was the revelation that the fall of humanity came through the act of eating what God told Adam and Eve not to eat (Genesis 3). This was such an important revelation because I had not realized the connection between consumption and the fall. Adam and Eve ate the forbidden fruit, and sometimes we suffer from ailments simply because we eat things we should not eat. The good news is that we still have the power to change and be healed. While you may be dealing with one ailment or another, I do believe that changing your diet has the power to change the way you feel. Here is what Nutritionist Fabienne has to say about a few of these conditions.

High Blood Pressure:

Fabienne says, "If we eat more of a plant-based diet, blood pressure wouldn't be an issue." Many of Fabienne's clients who have suffered high blood pressure usually tell her that they are eating bananas for potassium in an effort to regulate their pressure. However, according to Fabienne, a banana is not sufficient to eradicate high blood pressure. She believes that green leafy vegetables should be the most important foods in our diets. "We need about three servings of vegetables a day, but many people are barely consuming one serving. Vegetables like kale, collards, dandelion, spinach, and broccoli are important for those with high blood pressure because they are high in both potassium and calcium. In addition to greens, fiber is also important because it helps to decrease fat absorption and is great for colon health."

Fabienne states that in order to reverse high blood pressure, doctors usually say, "You need to lose weight," but she says, "change your plate." She recommends "giving your body a vacation" by eating a plant-based diet for one month, and then continue with mostly fish and greens thereafter. She suggests that during this vacation month we eliminate fried foods, foods high in salt, sweets, and any other foods that are harmful to our bodies. In addition, Fabienne says that juicing will do wonders for our health, so she suggests juicing apples or oranges with dandelion to regulate our blood pressure.

Diabetes:

Diabetes is prevalent in many communities, and it has been Fabienne's mission to promote pre-diabetes prevention, as well as help to facilitate healing in individuals who are diagnosed with the disease. Fabienne not only recommends eating a lot of greens, but she also suggests eating fish, such as wild sockeye salmon and sardines. In addition, it is highly recommended that individuals decrease their sugar intake. For those with Type 2 diabetes, Fabienne says the order in which you consume food is also important. "If you eat carbs first, before consuming protein and vegetables, you won't give your body enough time to produce insulin because of digestive system issues. So, by eating your protein and vegetables first, and then eating carbohydrates last, you will give your body enough time to produce the insulin that you need." It is also very important to avoid drinking juices filled with sugar and preservatives. Homemade tea and fresh juices mixed with dandelion are better alternatives. All in all, water is the best beverage.

Infertility:

Infertility is a very sensitive subject, one that many women have struggled with. I have a few friends who have had to deal with the physical and emotional trauma of the condition. It was important for me to highlight infertility and include Fabienne's expert advice because she has helped many of her clients conquer the condition.

Led by the Spirit of God, Fabienne received divine revelation from God regarding natural remedies for pregnancy. It was due to this revelation that Fabienne was able to give birth to three children—one while she was in her late 30s and two after the age of 40. When she was pregnant, God told her to take Coenzyme Q10. When she researched it, she discovered that it is a key vitamin for the cells, and specifically good for egg/reproductive health. To combat infertility Fabienne suggests combining the Coenzyme Q10 supplement, along with a tailored diet.

You may not be suffering from high blood pressure, diabetes or infertility, but you may be battling another ailment. Either way, you can assist in your own healing process by including natural remedies and changing your diet. Try scheduling a consultation with a nutritionist. They can guide you to the right natural remedy for your body type and condition. But, in addition to a nutritionist, begin taking small steps on your own toward your healing.

STEPS TO BEGIN A HEALTHIER REGIMEN

How do we begin the work of taking care of our bodies from a practical standpoint? It starts with making small changes until they become a new lifestyle. Start by making an assessment of your daily intake of food, as well as the amount of exercise you do. Once you have completed your assessment, begin to pray and ask God for wisdom to make the right decisions concerning the best foods to eat. My suggestion for small changes to your diet includes: drinking more water, eating more vegetables and fruits, and eating less sugar and salty foods. The goal is to replenish the nutrients that your body is lacking. While prayer is key, as previously mentioned, a nutritionist or health coach is also a great resource to help you on your journey to a healthier lifestyle.

In addition, while I recommend more walking, stretching and taking stairs instead of elevators or escalators, I also suggest consulting a personal trainer who will be able to provide guidance for the right exercises for your current physical condition. Small changes done on a consistent basis becomes a lifestyle. When we start to feel and see results, it encourages us to do more, and become a better version of ourselves. A healthier mind and body are what we all desire, but everything must be done in moderation. A healthier lifestyle does not mean crash dieting, or permanently excluding your favorite foods. Enjoy your tasty treats from time to time. Enjoy that piece of chocolate from time to time. Enjoy your favorite cake from time to time...but only *from time to time*. Moderation and balance are vital to maintaining your new healthy regimen.

No man is an island and God sends people to help us, teach us, and encourage us in life. We thank God for physicians who are qualified to evaluate our health conditions, and so scheduling regular examinations, as well as adhering to your doctor's advice, will put you on your path to healing. God gives us wisdom, and so we may need to take medications as a part of the healing process, but as believers, our faith is not in the medication, but in God. Jesus is the true Physician, and the true source of our complete healing and restoration. Man-made medications are helpful, but true healing comes from our spiritual medicine—the Word of God.

What steps can you take today to begin a healthier regimen?

_____

_____

_____

_____

_____

_____

_____

_____

_____

_____

_____

_____

_____

_____

_____

_____

_____

_____

Maintain

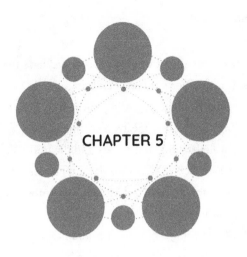

CHAPTER 5

Your Prescription

My child, be attentive to my words; incline your ear to my sayings. Do
not let them escape from your sight; keep them within your heart. For
they are life to those who find them, and healing to all their flesh.
— Proverbs 4:20-22 (NIV)

I t is said that a Proverb a day makes us wiser, and Godly wisdom is
imperative to believing, receiving, and maintaining our healing.
In this book of Proverbs, God uses King Solomon to instruct his
people, and it is in Proverbs 4:20–22 that God provides for us,
His people, our spiritual prescription. "My child, be attentive to
my words; incline your ear to my sayings. Do not let them escape
from your sight; keep them within your heart. For they are life to
those who find them, and healing to all their flesh" (NRSV). The

scripture calls us to attend to God's Word—to hide them within our hearts. It is the Word of God that brings life, but it is also the Word that brings healing. According to the Blue Letter Bible, the word "Healing" in the text means medicine, a cure, deliverance, remedy[9]—it is a refreshing of the body and the mind. God's Word is our spiritual medicine. When we pay attention to the Word of God, when we listen to the Word intently and embed them in our hearts—meditating on scripture, allowing it to take root in our hearts, we will yield a wellspring of life and healing in our bodies. The prescription is clear and healing is possible. Unlike man-made medicines, there are no negative side-effects for God's spiritual remedy. God's written Word is spiritual medicine that cures and delivers us from all infirmities. It refreshes our body and soul, it gives us hope, it transforms us, and it heals us from the inside out, and the only side-effect that occurs is a fortified faith.

God prescribes His Word as our spiritual medicine. Look up scriptures that speak to healing, stress, anxiety, or anything that may adversely affect your body. Once you have these specific scriptures, start consuming them. To consume means that you take the time to chew on God's Word—dissecting it, breaking it down, understanding it's meaning, and allowing it to penetrate your heart. Chew on it day and night, and pray with them fervently. To get you started, I have provided a list of scriptural medicine. Choose the ones that speak to your heart, then read them, pray with them, and meditate on them day and night. Take this spiritual medicine for as long as necessary (a week, a month, a year, etc.)—you can never overdose. Welcome the Holy Spirit in this process. Ask Him to lead during your meditation and prayer time. Here are some spiritual medicines accompanied by a prayer:

Psalm 41:3 (NIV)

"The LORD sustains them on their sickbed and restores them from their bed of illness."

Prayer: *Lord God, the all-sufficient God who sustains us on our sickbed and restores us from illness, please see about me in my condition and do for me the same as the writer of Psalm 41:3 declares. Lord, sustain me as I endure the healing process and restore me from this bed of illness, that I may be healed and made whole, in the name of Jesus I pray.*

Psalm 103:1–5 (NIV)

"Praise the LORD, my soul; all my inmost being, praise his holy name. Praise the LORD, my soul, and forget not all his benefits— who forgives all your sins and heals all your diseases, who redeems your life from the pit and crowns you with love and compassion, who satisfies your desires with good things so that your youth is renewed like the eagle's."

Prayer: *Lord, I praise you with my soul and all my innermost being. I praise your holy name! I praise you Lord with all of me and I take this time to remember all the benefits that come with being your child and loving you. Lord, I remember your gift of forgiveness. Thank you* *for forgiving me for all my sins of which I am truly sorry. Lord, I remember that you heal all our diseases and I thank you for the gift of healing, which I receive today by faith, in the name of Jesus Christ! Lord, I thank you for redeeming my life from the pit and crowning me with your love and compassion. Lord God, satisfy my desires with good things, with your complete healing, so that my youth is renewed like the eagles', in the name of Jesus I pray!*

Proverbs 3:7–8 (NRSV)

"Do not be wise in your own eyes; fear the LORD, and turn away from evil. It will be a healing for your flesh and a refreshment for your body."

Prayer: *Dear Lord, today I surrender my will to you, and I say "yes" to your will for my life. I choose not to be wise in my own eyes but I trust you, for you are the all-knowing, true, and living God. I decide this day to turn away from evil, in thought, word, and action. So now Lord, I receive your healing and refreshment for my body, in the name of Jesus!*

Isaiah 53:4–5 (NIV)

"Surely, he took up our pain and bore our suffering, yet we considered him punished by God, stricken by him, and afflicted. But he was pierced for our transgressions, he was crushed for our iniquities; the punishment that brought us peace was on him, and by his wounds we are healed."

Prayer: *Dear Heavenly Father, thank you for giving your son, my*

Lord and Savior, Jesus Christ to die on the cross as a living sacrifice for me. I thank you Lord Jesus for bearing my sickness/disease on the cross, and carrying my pain and sorrow so that I may be whole and set free. Lord, how grateful I am that you endured affliction for me, and allowed yourself to be wounded and bruised for all my sins. So, I thank you Father for the blood of Jesus, and today I declare that by His wounds I am healed and I am whole, in the name of Jesus!

Mark 5:25–29 (NIV)

"And a woman was there who had been subject to bleeding for twelve years. She had suffered a great deal under the care of many doctors and had spent all she had, yet instead of getting better she grew worse. When she heard about Jesus, she came up behind him in the crowd and touched his cloak, because she thought, 'If I just touch his clothes, I will be healed.' Immediately her bleeding stopped and she felt in her body that she was freed from her suffering."

Prayer: *Dear Heavenly Father, you know how long I've suffered, and like the woman with the issue of blood, I stretch forth my faith to touch the hem of Jesus' garment. Today I believe, by faith that as I touch Jesus, I am healed. I believe by faith that I am free from suffering. By faith I believe, and I thank you Lord for healing, in the name of Jesus!*

Mark 11:22–24 (NIV)

"'Have faith in God,' Jesus answered. 'Truly I tell you, if anyone says to this mountain, 'Go, throw yourself into the sea,' and does not doubt in their heart but believes that what they say will happen, it will be done for them. Therefore I tell you, whatever you ask for in prayer, believe that you have received it, and it will be yours."

Prayer: *Lord God, I choose to have faith in you! Lord I pray this prayer in faith according to Mark 11:23, and I speak to this mountain of illness (say the name of it) and I command it to leave my body now in Jesus' name. I command it to throw itself far away from me, and never return again. I believe by faith that it is done in the name of Jesus!*

Luke 5:12–13 (NKJV)

"And it happened when He was in a certain city, that behold, a man who was full of leprosy saw Jesus; and he fell on his face and implored Him, saying, 'Lord, if You are willing, You can make me clean.' Then He put out His hand and touched him, saying, 'I am willing; be cleansed.' Immediately the leprosy left him."

Prayer: *"Lord Jesus, you are no respecter of persons, and so just as you did for the man full of leprosy in Luke 5:12-13, I believe it is your will for me to be cleansed from this sickness (say the name of it). Lord I thank you for your love, and your willingness to heal me. I thank you Lord that by faith my body and mind are healed. I thank you for cleaning and delivering me in Jesus' name!"*

Luke 18:35–43 (MSG)

"He came to the outskirts of Jericho. A blind man was sitting beside the road asking for handouts. When he heard the rustle of the crowd, he asked what was going on. They told him, "Jesus the Nazarene is going by." He yelled, "Jesus! Son of David! Mercy, have mercy on me!" Those ahead of Jesus told the man to shut up, but he only yelled all the louder, "Son of David! Mercy, have mercy on me!" Jesus stopped and ordered him to be brought over. When he had come near, Jesus asked, "What do you want from me?" He said, "Master, I want to see again." Jesus said, "Go ahead—see again! Your faith has saved and healed you!" The healing was instant: He looked up, seeing—and then followed Jesus, glorifying God. Everyone in the street joined in, shouting praise to God."

Prayer: *"Lord, as the blind man cried out to you, I cry out to you Lord Jesus, have mercy on me! Lord Jesus, have mercy on me! Heal me and deliver me from this sickness (say the name of it). Lord, I believe that nothing is too hard for you. Lord, you are my help. You are my hope. You are my Healer. I believe you for healing in my body, mind and spirit! Make me whole Lord! Have mercy on me in Jesus' name!*

1 John 5:14–15 (NKJV)

"Now this is the confidence that we have in Him, that if we ask anything according to His will, He hears us. And if we know that He hears us, whatever we ask, we know that we have the petitions that we have asked of Him."

Prayer: *"Lord God, I believe it is your will that I be healed, so I am confident that you have heard my prayers to be healed from (say the name of the sickness/disease). Lord, according to 1 John 5:14-15, I thank you that you have already answered my prayers. I believe that*

I am free to live life abundantly and in good health. Lord, thank you that you are still a miracle-working God and that I am healed mentally, physically and spiritually, in the name of Jesus!"

Write your own prescription — scriptures and prayers

_____

_____

_____

_____

_____

_____

_____

_____

_____

_____

_____

_____

_____

_____

_____

_____

_____

_____

_____

_____

_____

_____

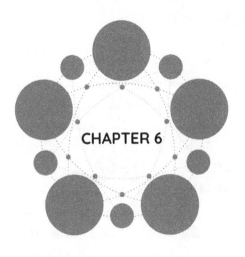

CHAPTER 6

The Network

Beloved, I pray that all may go well with you and that you may be in
good health, just as it is well with your soul.
— 3 John 1:2 (NRSV)

There is no quick fix, or a single action that will result in the total healing and restoration of a person. Healing requires a network. A network, according to Merriam-Webster Dictionary is an "interconnected or interrelated chain, group, or system" or an "informally interconnected group or association of persons (such as friends or professional colleagues)."[10] As believers seeking to be made whole, it is important that we create a healing network—an interconnection of faith, action, and relationships (The F.A.R principle) in order to believe, receive, and maintain our healing.

It takes faith, relationship with God, our connections to our fellow beings, prayer, and practical actions to maintain a physically, mentally, and spiritually healthy life. Our faith is the foundation of the healing network. It is on faith that every other component stands. Faith is the belief in God, in His love for us, in His Word and in His will for our lives. What does God's Word say about you? What does the Bible say about your condition? Whose report will you believe? Faith believes in the midst of pain. Faith strengthens us when we feel weak. It is faith—our unrelenting belief that God desires for us to be made whole that keeps us going day after day. God has called us to live by faith and not by sight. The trick of the enemy is to have us believe what we see and feel, but God calls us to move beyond our natural senses, and move into the supernatural—to believe God for the miraculous, and to have faith for the uncommon. God is able and is willing to heal you, but you must first believe.

Faith is living a life surrendered to God, and in obedience to God's will. Obedience calls us to action. Action is a major component of the healing network. What we do, and do not do, will have a direct impact on our healing process, whether negatively or positively. Our actions will reflect on our physical, spiritual and emotional wellbeing. Believing, receiving and maintaining our healing requires faith-inspired actions. This includes developing and sustaining an active prayer life. God calls us to pray without ceasing (1 Thessalonians 5:17). It includes making the decision to renew our minds by studying God's Word on a daily basis. We are called to meditate on the Word of God day and night (Psalm 1:2). We are called to have a positive frame of mind which yields a life of peace (Philippians 4:8-9). Our faith-inspired actions mean we are actively seeking God's presence and being intentional about our faith formation. Faith without works is dead (James 2:17), but the actions we take must be spiritual as well as practical.

Faith-inspired practical actions mean being intentional about caring for our minds and bodies. How are you eating and how are you living? Our bodies are the temple of God, and when we take care of it, we honor and glorify the Creator (1 Corinthians 6:19–20). God created the body to heal itself and he created food to sustain it. We are what we consume. Taking the steps to change our diets—to choose the right foods, to eat the seed-bearing plants given to us by God for nutrition and longevity (Genesis 1:29), to be disciplined to choose healthy alternatives—are vital to health and wholeness. Our faith-inspired actions within the healing network will allow us to see God's power working in our lives, but it is our relationships that form the supportive structure within the network.

How are you maintaining your relationships? Who is in your circle? Who are your confidants? Who are your prayer partners? Who needs to be removed from your inner circle? Who are your divine connections? What toxic relationships need to end? Who do you need to forgive? How strong is your relationship structure? We are created to be in relationship with God and with each other. Human beings have a natural desire for connection and human interactions. We need each other in order to not only live, but to thrive. In fact, in the beginning, God told Adam that it was not good for man (human being) to be alone, so He created man's helpmate in a woman named Eve (Genesis 2:18–25). We need each other and it is our relationships that bind us together and help us believe, receive and maintain our healing. So, what does your relationships within your network look like?

As you embark on this healing journey it will be necessary for you to evaluate the impact of your relationships. How are your connections helping or hurting you? Iron sharpens iron (Proverbs 27:17)—are you being sharpened? Developing a good supportive structure includes accountability partners, health professionals, spiritual mentors, prayer partners, and those good ol' friends who know you, genuinely love you and allow you to be you. Your health and healing are priority, so be discerning about who you allow in your space during this season of your life. Believing, receiving, and maintaining your healing requires a clean, wholesome, positive, faith-filled environment. Guard your space, and do not be afraid to remove anyone, and anything that does not contribute positively to your healing. I encourage you to pray for divine friendships, partnerships, mentors and teachers. The more divinely-connected relationships you maintain the stronger your supportive structure will be for an overall healthier lifestyle.

IN CONCLUSION:

"Beloved, I pray that all may go well with you and that you

may be in good health, just as it is well with your soul" (3 John 1:2 NRSV). This is my heart's prayer for you. I pray that you live a holistic lifestyle. Remember, The F.A.R. Principle, is the major components of your Healing Network. When all three components are in place and are working in conjunction with each other, then believing, receiving, and maintaining your healing is possible. Through Jesus, you can live the abundant life, lacking nothing. He died so that by His stripes you are healed (Isaiah 53:4-5). He died so that you can have the surpassing victory—you are more than a conqueror (Romans 8:37). Regardless of what it looks like, or feels like, you win! Sickness does not have the last word, but Jesus does! Work your healing network! Build and sustain your faith. Let your actions match your faith. Maintain your divine connections. Work your healing network! You can do it. You will do it, and declare that it's already done in your life. No matter what you are going through, no matter the diagnosis, God desires for you to be healed. Work your healing network! Believe, receive, and maintain your healing in Jesus' name!

Healed.

NOTES

CHAPTER 1:

1. Dictionary.com, s.v. "forever," accessed September 1, 2020 *https://www.dictionary.com/browse/forever*

2. Blue Letter Bible *https://www.blueletterbible.org/lang/Lexicon/ Lexicon.cfm?strongs=G386&t=KJV*

CHAPTER 2:

3. Kenneth E. Hagin. The Believer's Authority. Oklahoma: Rhema Bible Church, 1986. Pg. 33

CHAPTER 3:

4. Merriam-Webster Dictionary, s.v. "mountain," accessed September 1, 2020 *https://www.merriam-webster.com/dictionary/ mountain*

5. Gina Roberts-Grey, "Forgive! Why Your Life Could Depend On It," Essence Magazine, June 5, 2017. *https://www.essence. com/love-sex/relationships/forgive-your-life-could-depend-it/*

6. American Psychological Association, "Impact of Stress," 2012, *https://www.apa.org/news/press/releases/stress/2012/impact.aspx*

7. Mayo Clinic Team, "Positive thinking: Stop negative self-talk to reduce stress," June 9, 2011. *https://www.mayoclinic.org/ healthy-lifestyle/stress-management/in-depth/positive-thinking/ art-20043950*

CHAPTER 4

8. Rachael Link, MS, RD, "Alkaline Water: Beneficial or All Hype?," Draxe.com, October 4, 2018. *https://draxe.com/alkaline-water/*

CHAPTER 5

9. Blue Letter Bible *https://www.blueletterbible.org/lang/Lexicon/Lexicon.cfm?strongs=H4832&t=KJV*

CHAPTER 6

10. Merriam-Webster Dictionary, s.v. "network," accessed September 1, 2020. *https://www.merriam-webster.com/dictionary/network*